G. K. Khaira
Magdalen College
Oxford.

Introduction to clinical clerking

Introduction to

CLINICAL CLERKING

CAROL A. SEYMOUR

Lecturer in Medicine and Fellow of Trinity College
University of Cambridge

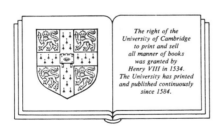

The right of the University of Cambridge to print and sell all manner of books was granted by Henry VIII in 1534. The University has printed and published continuously since 1584.

Cambridge University Press

Cambridge
London New York New Rochelle
Melbourne Sydney

Published by the Press Syndicate of the University of Cambridge
The Pitt Building, Trumpington Street, Cambridge CB2 1RP
32 East 57th Street, New York, NY 10022, USA
296 Beaconsfield Parade, Middle Park, Melbourne 3206, Australia

© Cambridge University Press 1984

First published 1984

Printed in Great Britain at the University Press, Cambridge

Library of Congress Catalogue card number: 84–45240

British Library Cataloguing in Publication Data
Seymour, Carol A.
Introduction to clinical clerking.

1. Medical history taking 2. Physical diagnosis
I. Title
616.07′51   RC65
ISBN 0 521 26552 5

WD

I keep six honest serving-men
(They taught me all I knew);
Their names are What and Why and When
And How and Where and Who.

(Rudyard Kipling: *Just-So Stories*, The Elephant's Child)

Contents

Preface

This is the second edition of this book which was devised specifically for clinical students just starting their 'clerkships'. It aims to provide a simple guide to history-taking and clinical examination during the initial introductory period of a clinical course and during the first medical and surgical attachments. It is only meant as a rough guide for students, who will eventually build up their own method of clinical examination based on their reading, experience and what is taught on the wards.

I am grateful to Dr Richard Page who helped me to prepare the first edition when he was Senior Registrar in the Department of Medicine at the University of Cambridge, and to Dr German Berrios of the Department of Psychiatry, University of Cambridge, who provided the basis of the section on taking a psychiatric history. I also wish to thank Mrs Glynis Moore for her painstaking typing and help in organising the book.

C.A.S.

Abbreviations

AS	Alimentary system
ASD	Atrial septal defect
BBB	Bundle branch block
b.d.s.	Twice a day
BP	Blood pressure
BS	Breath sounds
c̄	With (*cum*)
c/o	Complains of
CNS	Central nervous system
CVS	Cardiovascular system
CXR	Chest X-ray
ECG	Electrocardiograph
EOM	External ocular muscles
FE	Functional enquiry
FEV_1	Forced expiratory volume in 1 minute
FH	Family history
FVC	Forced vital capacity
GUS	Genito-urinary system
Hb	Haemoglobin
HPC	History of the present complaint
HS	Heart sounds
i.m.	Intramuscular
i.v.	Intravenous
JVP	Jugular venous pulse
LMN	Lower motor neurone lesion
MS	Locomotor system
OS	Opening snap
PDA	Patent ductus arteriosus
PERLA	Pupils equal, regular, react equally to light and accommodation
PH	Personal history
PMH	Past medical history
PN	Percussion note
POMR	Problem orientated medical record
PR	Rectal examination (*per rectum*)
PV	Vaginal examination (*per vaginam*)
q.d.s.	Four times a day
RS	Respiratory system

s̄   Without (*sine*)
SH   Social history
SOB Shortness of breath
t.d.s. Three times a day
TVF Tactile vocal fremitus
UMN Upper motor neurone lesion
VSD Ventricular septal defect
WBC White blood cell count

Introduction

This booklet aims to provide students at the beginning of their clinical course with a scheme for taking a history and performing a physical examination. It is not suggested that the scheme is followed rigidly, as the various medical specialities place different emphases on different parts of the history and examination, but rather that it should form a framework upon which to build. Throughout the booklet there are notes on the interpretation of various findings and suggestions for writing up case notes. The blank page on the left is for the student to write annotations to the text. By the end of the first medical or surgical attachment, these notes, compiled by the student, should represent more accurately the student's individual system for clinical clerking. At the back of the booklet there is a specimen history, with an account of how Problem Orientated Medical Records are constructed and a checklist that should be used whilst clerking a patient. A scheme for taking a psychiatric history and assessing the mental state of a patient is also included.

To get the most out of the clerkship, it is important that patients are seen as soon as possible after their admission and that the clerking is done without reference to the House Officer's notes. Thereafter these patients should be seen at least once a day and the case notes kept thoroughly up to date. Only by seeing numerous patients in the acute phase of their illness and formulating one's own ideas about them, can any skill and fluency in clerking patients be acquired.

Finally, it should never be forgotten that illness is usually unpleasant and very often frightening for the patient and that the development of a sensitive and professional approach to the patient is as important as the acquisition of clinical acumen.

Scheme for taking a case history

History
Physical examination
Summary of positive findings
Provisional or differential diagnosis
Special investigations
Progress notes
Discharge note
Final diagnosis

The history

The aim of the history is to obtain a complete picture of the patient's present condition which is then interpreted in the light of their past history, family history, occupation, habits and social circumstances. If the patient is unable to give an adequate or reliable history then the necessary information must be obtained from other sources (which should be stated) such as friends, relatives or ambulance men, and you should therefore arrange with the House Officer to be present when these sources are interviewed. This is particularly important when the patient is admitted in a coma or following a bout of unconsciousness (e.g. epileptic fit), when a description of the event by an eye-witness may be of considerable diagnostic value.

The record of the history and examination needs to be concise and in addition to documenting all positive information, it should contain statements about relevant negative data. Notes should be prefaced by your name and the date of the interview and should be written in headed sections. By convention the history may be taken, and is recorded, in the following order:

Presenting complaint   (c/o)
History of the present complaint   (HPC)
Past medical history   (PMH)
Family history   (FH)
Personal and social history   (PH and SH)
Drugs and allergy history
Functional enquiry   (FE)
  General
  Cardiovascular system   (CVS)
  Respiratory system   (RS)
  Alimentary system   (AS)
  Genito-urinary system   (GUS)
  Central nervous system   (CNS)
  Endocrine system
  Locomotor system

Basic data (personal details)

The interview should begin by introducing yourself to the patient.
Then note:

> Name
> Address
> Age
> Sex
> Occupation
> Date of admission (date when patient actually clerked)
> Nature of admission (i.e. routine or emergency)
> Name of General Practitioner
>> (you should always refer to the General Practitioner by name whenever possible and not simply as 'your GP')

Example
Mr X, 1 Florence Way, Cambridge. Age 56 years, a baker. Admitted to Y ward at 4 p.m. on 12.7.83 (as emergency or routine admission) under the care of Dr Z (or Mr Z).

Presenting complaint (c/o)

When you have gained the patient's confidence, identify the major symptoms and their duration by asking:

> 1. 'What is the main problem as far as you are concerned?'
or 2. 'What are your main symptoms?'
or 3. 'What has brought you into hospital?'

It is important that the patient's *major symptoms* are recorded simply and not his/her or someone else's interpretation of them. This preliminary information is usually given as:
Complains of (c/o):

> 1. Shortness of breath on exertion for six months (6/12)
> 2. Ankle swelling for 1 week (1/52)
> 3. Retrosternal chest pain for 1 day (1/7)

not: The patient complains of dyspnoea, oedema or heart disease.

Further details of these problems should be recorded in the next section (HPC).
NB: Other major problems may become evident at a later stage of the history-taking and these should subsequently be added to this list of major complaints.

History of the present complaint (HPC)

The history of the present complaint should begin by stating when the patient was last perfectly well. It should continue with the onset of any symptoms, which should then be described in chronological order, noting both the actual date of onset and the duration. (Symptoms should never be dated by the day of the week as this rapidly becomes meaningless.)

Then follows a detailed description of each symptom, and for this purpose the patient's own words should be used where possible and whenever relevant. It must be emphasised that *all* symptoms must be described in detail whether they seem relevant or not.

It is totally unrealistic to expect patients to give a succinct and dated account of the development of their symptoms in chronological order. You will therefore find it necessary to ask a number of questions, which should be phrased in such a way that the answer is not suggested by the question, and to rearrange the story in chronological order.

Many patients will need guidance from such questions as:

When were you last well?

What was the first thing you noticed?

Do you remember clearly the first occasion you had the pain, headache, dizziness, etc.?

What were you doing at the time?

Have any other symptoms occurred since then and, if so, in what order did they occur?

Have the original symptoms persisted or disappeared and have others taken their place?

What troubles you most at the moment?

Have you noticed anything that makes you better or worse?

Have you received any treatment? What effect has it had?

What do you think is the cause of all the trouble?

Have you been able to work since the trouble began and, if not, why not?

History of the present complaint should include:

Chronology of symptoms

Elaboration of symptoms

Relevant questions from functional enquiry for the appropriate system (e.g. CVS: see p. 12)

Certain symptoms are so important that they require special analysis. For example:

Cough

Character	– Tickle in throat or from chest; painful or easy
Sputum	– From throat or chest; quantity; colour; haemoptysis; viscidity
Time	– Continuous or intermittent; association with work, time of day or night; chronicity (recurrent each year and lasting 3/12 may indicate chronic bronchitis)
Contributory causes	– Cold; exercise; posture
Associated phenomena	– Wheezing; pain; vomiting
Procedures which relieve cough	

Shortness of breath (SOB)

Character	– True shortness of breath; audible wheezing or sensation that breathing is difficult
Time	– Continuous, intermittent or paroxysmal; association with seasons, work, time of day or night (paroxysmal nocturnal dyspnoea is shortness of breath at night)
Contributory causes	– Exercise (quantitative statement of amount of exercise required to elicit dyspnoea); cough-ing; excitement; pain; relationship to lying flat (orthopnoea); how many pillows?
Associated phenomena	– Wheezing; pain; palpitation or other symptoms
Procedures which relieve breathlessness	

Palpitations

Frequency and duration of attacks; relation to exercise, meals, coffee and other symptoms; sensation of dropped beats; sudden or gradual start and finish; pulse rate during the episode (ask patient to tap out the rate).

Character	– Effortless; regurgitation; projectile; self-induced; nausea; straining
Vomitus	– Quantity; colour; constituents; haematemesis (altered blood has appearance of 'coffee grounds')
Time	– Frequency; time of day or night
Contributory causes	– Meals; coughing; drug ingestion
Associated phenomena	– Pain; sweating; shivering

Relief of other symptoms by vomiting

Indigestion

| Character | – Determine what the patient means by indigestion; e.g. loss of appetite; flatulence; heartburn; regurgitation; feeling of fullness; nausea; vomiting; abdominal pain |
| Associated phenomena | – Meals, particular foods; constipation, or other symptoms |

Procedures which relieve indigestion

Diarrhoea

Character	– Urgency; incontinence
Stools	– Consistency; colour; mucus; blood; odour (offensive suggests steatorrhoea or melaena)
Time	– Frequency and time of day or night
Associated phenomena	– Pain; tenesmus (continual inclination to void the rectum, accompanied by painful straining)

Pain

A full analysis of this symptom is important and the following features should be sought:

| Location | – Site of maximum intensity (describe in terms of surface anatomy); distribution and radiation (note where pain is first felt and to where it spreads when at its height) |
| Character | – Knife-like, stabbing; colicky; aching; gnawing; dragging; is it real pain or merely discomfort? |

Severity	– Does it cause the patient to 'double up'? In a woman who has had children, compare with labour pains. Degree of incapacity (Can you work with the pain? Can you keep still? Is there sweating or vomiting?)
Time	– When pain first began; mode of onset and of ending; the duration of attack; frequency; continuous or intermittent; relation to day or night
Associated symptoms	– Nausea; vomiting

Any factors known to produce or relieve the pain

Past medical history (PMH)

The past medical history should include an account of *all* previous illnesses or operations, whether apparently important or not. The patient is first given the opportunity to recall past illnesses and then certain events are enquired for specifically by questions such as: 'Have you ever been "off work", admitted to hospital or undergone an operation?'

If the patient has had illnesses or operations in the past, note the date and whether recovery was uncomplicated. Some idea of the severity may be gained by asking how long the patient was in bed and/or away from work. In doubtful cases do not accept the 'diagnosis' of the patient, but ask the patient to describe the illness and form your own conclusion. It is often helpful to enquire whether the patient has ever had a general medical examination in the past and if so whether he or she was pronounced fit (if in the Forces, ask if discharged A1).

All past complaints should be recorded in chronological order:

Childhood illnesses	– Rheumatic fever (recurrent tonsillitis, 'growing pains'); measles, etc.
Other illnesses	– Diabetes; jaundice; tuberculosis. (Drugs, and if so for how long; surgery)
Operations	– Note relevant details and complications
Accidents	– Did these occur by chance or were they related to occupation?
Pregnancies	– Include number, live and dead births, and complications.

Family history (FH)

The purpose of taking a family history is to obtain evidence of similar disease in other members of the family. Some diseases are clearly inherited in a dominant or recessive fashion whereas in others it is a susceptibility that appears to be inherited (e.g. diabetes mellitus). Additionally, clustering of disease in families may indicate the same causal agent. A further reason for taking the family history is that it could reveal illnesses which may affect the patient in the future.

Ask whether there has been any illness in the family, such as diabetes, heart disease, hypertension, peptic ulcers. Record the state of health of all relatives and, if any relative has died, state at what age and ascertain the cause tactfully.

Minimal statement of family history

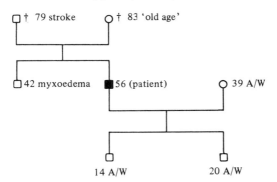

or:	Father	†79	stroke
	Mother	†83	'old age'
	1 Brother	42	myxoedema
	Wife	39	A/W
	2 Sons	14/20	A/W

No hypertension or heart disease
No diabetes or thyroid disease

Abbreviations

†	dead	■	patient
□	male	A/W	alive and well
○	female		

Personal and social history (PH and SH)

The personal and social history should provide a picture of the patient's background, occupation, home environment, worries, personality, and alcohol and tobacco consumption. Much of it may have already been established during the course of the history taking, but if not further specific details should be sought.

Alcohol and tobacco consumption

Present and past occupations. Note particularly the nature of the job and whether there is or was any occupational hazard, e.g. exposure to dusts or chemicals.

Circumstances and conditions at home. These may be relevant to the patient's admission and are very relevant to the patient's discharge from hospital (e.g. whether there are stairs, outside toilet). Mention should also be made of any pets, such as dogs or pigeons.

Recent travel. Note countries visited.

Further information. When indicated, further information such as education, domestic and financial worries or sexual history may be helpful.

Minimal statement of personal and social history

Smokes 25 cigarettes per day, alcohol socially only
Baker for 30 years – flour dust + +
Lives with wife and two sons in their own home
No social or financial problems

Drugs and allergy history

It is important to enquire for known allergies:

Do you have any allergies, such as eczema or asthma?
Have you ever had a reaction to a drug?

It is also important to document exactly what treatment the patient is taking at the time (and its duration) and other treatments recently stopped. For example:

Digoxin 0.25 mg daily for several years
Ampicillin 250 mg q.d.s. for the last 4/7
Finished a 10/7 course of Oxytetracycline 4/7 ago

Minimal statement of drugs and allergy history

No allergies
Taking no therapy ($R = 0$)

Functional enquiry (FE)

The major purpose of the functional enquiry is to unearth symptoms of which the patient has not complained spontaneously. Since the lack of certain symptoms as well as their presence is often helpful in diagnosis, these questions are asked in every case and the answer recorded whether positive or negative. Many of the questions may already have been asked during the history of the present complaint and clearly should not be repeated. If significant symptoms are identified during this enquiry, further details are then sought and recorded under the appropriate section (e.g. History of the Present Complaint and Past Medical History).

In the scheme that follows, the questions that are asked routinely are given on the left-hand side of the page under their appropriate system headings, and examples of further questions which may be relevant in certain circumstances on the right-hand side of the page.

Routine questions	**Additional questions if indicated**

General

Fatigue	– Pyrexias; rigors; sweats
General malaise	
Sleep disturbance	– Difficulty in getting to sleep; early waking
Weight loss or gain	– How much and over what time? do clothes still fit?
Skin lesions	– Rashes; bruising (purpura) Bleeding tendencies

Cardiovascular system (CVS)

Shortness of breath	– Duration; exercise tolerance; orthopnoea; paroxysmal nocturnal dyspnoea
Chest pain	– Duration; character; radiation; relationship to exertion or respiration
Palpitations	– Frequency; duration of attacks; whether they start and stop suddenly; pulse rate during attack; provoking or relieving factors; regular or irregular
Swelling of legs	– Duration; whether present after a night's rest; presence of varicose veins

Respiratory system (RS)

Shortness	– As in
of breath	CVS
Chest pain	– Increased by respiration, e.g. pleuritic
Cough	– Duration; first thing in the morning or all day; association with smoking
Sputum	– Amount (e.g. eggcupfuls); colour
Haemoptysis	– Duration; whether frank blood or mixed with sputum; relationship to bad coughing bout; associated chest pain
Wheezing	

Alimentary system (AS)

Appetite	– Normal or reduced; if reduced, is it associated with weight loss?
Sore mouth/	– Presence of aphthous
tongue	ulcers
Difficulty in	– Dysphagia for foods, for solids; site where food
swallowing	sticks
Acid	– Bitter taste in mouth
regurgitation	(water brash)
Indigestion	– Location; any flatulence
Nausea and	– Haematemesis (frank blood or 'coffee
vomiting	grounds')
Abdominal	– Duration; site; relationship to meals, posture,
pains	bowels, micturition, etc.
Bowel	– Regular or irregular; diarrhoea (frequency,
frequency	day and/or night, consistency, associated blood or mucus, melaena (black tarry motions)); constipation (duration, how often bowels opened, when last opened, associated pain)

Genito-urinary system (GUS)

Micturition	– Dysuria (i.e. pain on micturition); frequency; polyuria; polydipsia (Are your waterworks all right?)
Symptoms of	– Difficulty in starting micturition;
prostatism	poor stream; terminal dribble;
(older men)	nocturia

(*continued overleaf*)

Nocturia — Duration; number of times

Haematuria

For men — Symptoms of prostatism

For women: menstruation

Age of onset (*K*) ⎫ Recorded as:
Periodicity   ⎬ Length of period
Regularity $K = 13 \dfrac{4\text{--}5 \ (\text{days})}{28 \ (\text{days})}$ regular, not heavy or
Light or heavy ⎭   painful (dysmenorrhoea)

Intermenstrual discharge

Menopause — Post-menopausal bleeding

Central nervous system (CNS)

Headache — Duration; frequency; site; intensity; wakes with it (suggests raised intracranial pressure); related to anxieties or reading; associated phenomena

Fits or faints — Duration; frequency; how long unconscious; associated incontinence; tongue biting or convulsion; aura

Vision — Glasses; general or specific impairment (scotomata or hemianopia); loss of vision

Hearing (deafness) — Duration; one or both ears; tinnitus; dizziness; vertigo

Weakness of limbs — Duration; progressive; unsteadiness of gait

Numbness or paraesthesiae — Duration; site; frequency; provoking position

Memory or personality change — Personality changes; apathetic; irritable
Loss of memory or concentration
Dysphasia or dysarthria
Right or left-handed
Smell, taste
Past history of head injury; aural/nasal infections

Locomotor system

Joints — Any pain, stiffness or swelling of the joints
Morning stiffness; duration

Weakness of limbs — As in CNS

Endocrine system

Irritability	
Thirst	– Polydipsia, polyuria (may indicate diabetes, pituitary abnormality)
Weather intolerance	– preference for hot/cold conditions (may indicate thyroid disease: hypothyroidism/ hyperthyroidism)
Hair	– Loss (alopecia: may indicate thyroid disease) or growth (hirsutism) of hair
	Disposition over body (may indicate pituitary or ovarian/testicular abnormality)

Minimal statement of the functional enquiry

(when no morbid symptoms are present)

This should include a statement about *every* question listed on the left-hand side of the page under each system (see checklist on pp. 71–2).

Scheme for the physical examination

The physical examination has several objectives:

1. To seek a physical cause for the patient's symptoms and if possible assess its nature, extent and severity.
2. To obtain objective evidence of apparent normality as well as abnormality in the various parts of the body.
3. To screen for abnormalities of which the patient may be unaware and which may be totally unrelated to the presenting condition (e.g. hypertension, rectal carcinoma).

Suggested scheme for approaching the examination of a patient

At all stages to ensure the patient's privacy and comfort. Explain to the patient what you are going to do, both initially and again at appropriate stages of the examination.

Since the examination of the individual systems (described in detail later) is rarely conducted rigidly system by system, the following scheme is given as a guideline:

1. If possible start the examination with the patient fully clothed, sitting comfortably in bed at an angle of 45°.
2. Make a general assessment of how well or ill the patient appears and note any obvious abnormalities.
3. Examine the pulse and hands, particularly the nails; compare radial and brachial pulses on the two sides. Feel for epitrochlear gland enlargement and note any joint abnormalities.
4. Examine the head and neck, paying attention to the hair, mucous membranes, tongue, teeth, thyroid and neck lymphadenopathy.
5. Having gained the patient's confidence, ask him/her to remove his/her clothing to expose the chest, but make sure that the abdomen and legs remain covered. Now examine cardiorespiratory systems as described later. Finally examine the breasts (mainly applies to female patients) and axillae, note any muscle wasting in the upper limbs and then allow the patient to cover the upper half.
6. Then examine the abdomen (keeping the genital region covered), the groins for lymphadenopathy and check the

hernial orifices. Look for delay between radial and femoral pulses if appropriate (e.g. dissecting aneurysm, coarctation of aorta). *Always* leave a rectal or genital examination until the rest of the examination is completed.

7. The examination of the nervous system begins with an assessment of 'higher centres' and an examination of the cranial nerves.
8. Next examine the upper limbs for wasting, power and reflexes, and (where relevant) sensation.
9. Then examine the lower limbs for the first time (keeping the genital region covered) and note any abnormalities of the skin, joints and pulses. Finally, examine for wasting, power, reflexes and (where appropriate) sensation.

By convention the examination is recorded as follows:

General
Cardiovascular system (CVS)
Respiratory system (RS)
Alimentary system (AS)
Central nervous system (CNS)
Locomotor system (MS)

In order to be clear, each system has been considered separately here. This involves some repetition, but as you gain experience the examination will become more integrated. It is, however, essential to be able to examine any of the systems separately.

Missing important signs or abnormalities is minimised by conducting the examination of any part of the body methodically. The conventional order is:

Inspection
Palpation
Percussion
Auscultation

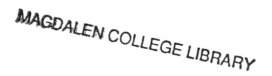

18

Examination of any lump or mass

The examination of any lump or mass can be used to illustrate the conventional order of examination:

Inspection	– Location of lump; colour; movement; pulsation; associated skin changes; trans-illumination (i.e. fluid-filled, air-filled or solid)
Palpation	– Situation; shape; size; consistency (including fluctuation); attachments; mobility; pulsation; can it be emptied? (e.g. hernia)
Percussion	– Resonant or dull (i.e. air-filled, fluid-filled or solid)
Auscultation	– Arterial or venous bruits; bowel sounds

19

General examination

Measurements on admission (this applies to emergency admissions)

Temperature
Pulse rate
Respiration rate
Blood pressure

General examination

The record of the general examination should be a word-picture
of the patient's general condition and include a statement about
certain abnormalities which are sought in every case. It is *not*,
therefore, limited to the initial observations of the patient.

General condition	– Well/ill; comfortable/in pain; breathless; feverish
Physical appearance	– Thin; fat; evidence of recent weight loss; dehydration (inelastic skin, dry tongue)
Position in bed	– Propped up; lying flat comfortably; restless, etc.
Mental state	– Alert; drowsy; confused; cooperative
Nutrition	– Obese; wasted; thin
Skin	– Complexion; pallor; cyanosis; jaundice; pigmentation; rashes; striae (purple abdominal stretch marks); spider naevi and palmar erythema (cutaneous stigmata of liver disease)
Mucous membranes	– Pale or good colour; pigmentation
Nails	– Clubbing koilonychia (spoon-shaped); splinter haemorrhages (splinter-like lesions under nails suggesting bacterial endocarditis)
Hair	– Texture; loss of hair from head (alopecia); hirsutism premature greying (pernicious anaemia)
Breath odour	– Smell of ketones (in ketoacidosis); alcohol
Eyes	– Colour of sclerae; exophthalmos or enophthalmos
Neck	– Abnormal lymph nodes; venous engorgement; pulsation or tumours
Thyroid gland	– Inspect and palpate; note movement on swallowing; presence of mass or bruit

20

Examination of the lymphatic system

Examine neck for enlarged lymph nodes, including pre-auricular, post-auricular, submental, submandibular, superficial and deep cervical, occipital and subclavian regions. In addition feel for Virchow's node behind lower insertion or sternomastoid (associated with carcinoma of stomach).

Examine epitrochlear (sarcoid or syphilis), axillary and groin regions (inguinal nodes should be palpated as part of the abdominal examination).

Look for enlargement of veins at the root of the neck or front of the chest indicative of mediastinal glandular enlargement. The glands of the posterior abdominal wall should be carefully palpated when examining the abdomen (will be enlarged e.g. when testicular tumours are present).

Examination of the breast

Inspection	– Shape and symmetry
	– Obvious mass, redness or *peau d'orange* (an orange skin appearance seen occasionally in carcinoma of the breast)
	– Nipple retraction; discharge, clear, milky, blood-stained; eczema
Palpation	– Site; localised or multiple diffuse lumps; tenderness (note the quadrant of the breast)
	– If lumps are found, examine the axillary lymph nodes very thoroughly

Minimal statement of the general examination

(when no morbid signs exist)

Healthy looking, well nourished
Afebrile
No anaemia
No cyanosis
No jaundice
Thyroid not enlarged
No clubbing
No lymphadenopathy
Breasts normal

21

Examination of the cardiovascular system

The presence or absence of shortness of breath, cyanosis, clubbing, oedema and stigmata of hyperlipidaemia (e.g. corneal arcus or xanthelasmata) will have been noted during the general examination and if not should always be ascertained in an examination of the cardiovascular system.

Pulse

Note rate, rhythm, volume and character (from palpation of brachial or carotid arteries).

Rhythm	– Irregularly irregular (rate and volume) (e.g. atrial fibrillation)
	– Accelerating on inspiration, slowing on expiration ($=$ sinus arrhythmia)
	– Dropped beats (e.g. ectopic beats)
Volume	– Weak thready pulse – in hypotension
Character	– Small volume; slow rising or plateau pulse (e.g. aortic stenosis)
	– Rapid 'upstroke' and 'downstroke', i.e. water hammer pulse (e.g. aortic regurgitation, any hyperdynamic circulatory state)
	– Weakening or disappearance with inspiration $=$ pulsus paradoxus (when systolic blood pressure reduced by greater than 10 mm Hg) (e.g. constrictive pericarditis, haemo-pericardium)
Peripheral vessels	– The following pulses are sought in every patient and compared on the two sides (at the appropriate stage of examination): temporal, carotid, brachial, radial, femoral, popliteal, dorsalis pedis, posterior tibial (inequality between radial–radial or radial–femoral pulses may indicate coarctation of aorta or dissection of aorta)
	– Peripheral perfusion should be noted, i.e. whether limbs warm or cold, hair distribution
	– The presence of varicose veins should also be noted
Oedema	– Test for dependent oedema (pitting of skin with gentle pressure) over ankles, shins and sacrum

22

Blood pressure (BP)

Record arm used and whether lying (•≪), sitting (⚹), or standing (⚹). If relevant, note whether pressure varies with respiration or posture.
Measurement of BP:

Systolic   – Appearance of sounds
Diastolic   – Muffling of sounds (Koratkov IV)
                   – Disappearance of sounds (Koratkov V)

Where atrial fibrillation is present, take an average BP of several readings.

Jugular venous pulse (JVP)

When the patient is lying at an angle of 45° the sternal angle is an approximate surface marker of the right atrium. In normal subjects, the mean right atrial pressure is 2–3 cm of water and so, in this position, venous pulsation in the neck is barely visible.

If the neck veins are *engorged but non-pulsatile*, obstruction to their emptying by tumour or by compression in the cervical fascia is indicated.

If the neck veins are *engorged and pulsatile*, raised right atrial pressure is present.

If the neck veins *cannot be seen*, this implies *normal* or *low* right atrial pressure *or* that the neck veins are obscured by fat and muscle. If the veins can be seen to fill when compressed by a finger placed just above the clavicle, and to empty when the finger is removed, the right atrial pressure is not raised.

The jugular venous pulse has two components:

'a' wave   Atrial contraction
'v' wave   Atrial filling against closed tricuspid valve in late
                systole

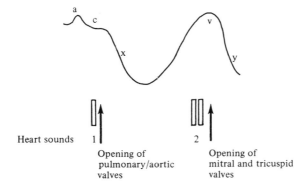

23

Heart sounds 1

Opening of
pulmonary/aortic
valves

Opening of
mitral and tricuspid
valves

a   Atrial contraction
c   Closure of tricuspid valve during ventricular systole
x   Descent as atria relax
v   Venous return whilst tricuspid valve is shut
y   Descent as tricuspid valve opens and blood rapidly
     enters right ventricle

Examples of raised JVP

Big 'a' wave   – Tricuspid or pulmonary stenosis
                – Pulmonary hypertension
                – Complete heart block
Absent 'a' wave– Atrial fibrillation
Big 'v' wave   – Tricuspid regurgitation

Examination of the heart

Inspection and palpation

The **position**, **force** and **character** of chest wall pulsations are the
most important guide to the size of the heart and its various
chambers.

1. **Apex beat.** This is the outermost and lowest pulsation palpable
and is normally in the 5th intercostal space internal to the mid-
clavicular line.

Displacement of apex beat

    Congenital, e.g. skeletal abnormalities, dextrocardia
    Extrinsic, e.g. tension pneumothorax ('pushed over')
                pulmonary fibrosis ('pulled over')

Intrinsic, e.g. ischaemic heart disease – left ventricular
hypertrophy as in mitral/aortic regurgi-
tation, left ventricular failure

24

(Cardiac enlargement or mediastinal displacement may affect the position of the apex beat.) Note its character and position and if abnormal measure it.

Changes in cardiac impulse

Left ventricular hypertrophy: Forceful heaving impulse
(e.g. aortic stenosis, systemic hypertension,
mitral and aortic incompetence)
Right ventricular hypertrophy: 'Parasternal heave' to left
of sternum (e.g. pulmonary hypertension)

(Left ventricular enlargement gives rise to a forceful heaving impulse displaced downwards and laterally. The apical impulse has a tapping quality in mitral stenosis.)

2. **Other impulses** (not seen or felt in health at rest)

Pulsation of the lower sternum and left costal cartilages:
Suggests right ventricular enlargement
Pulsation in the 2nd and 3rd left intercostal spaces:
Suggests pulmonary artery enlargement
Pulsation in the 2nd right intercostal space:
Suggests ascending aortic aneurysm
Double impulse at the apex:
Suggests ventricular aneurysm

3. **Thrills.** These are palpable murmurs and should be recorded.

Percussion

This is rarely helpful although used by some to assess cardiac size.

Auscultation

Time all cardiac events by palpating the carotid pulse at the same time as listening.

1. **Heart sounds (HS).** These are caused by valve closure.

First HS – mitral and tricuspid closure
Second HS – aortic (A) and pulmonary (P) closure

These are normally easily heard.

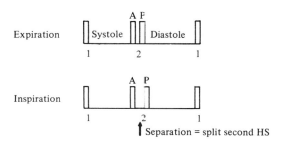

25

Note splitting of the HS (both components being audible):

First HS   – Normal

Right or left bundle branch block (BBB)

Second HS   – Normal

Right BBB if widely split and widens on inspiration

Atrial septal defect (ASD) if widely split and unaffected by inspiration (fixed)

Note loudness of the HS:

Loud first HS   – Mitral stenosis

Short P–R interval

Hyperdynamic circulation

Loud second HS

– Pulmonary component: pulmonary hypertension

Aortic component: systemic hypertension

Faint HS   – Thick chest wall

Emphysema

Stenotic or incompetent valves

Record the HS diagrammatically:

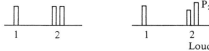

2. **Extra heart sounds.**

Third HS   – An early diastolic sound indicates heart disease in those over 25 years but is occasionally heard in young normal subjects

Fourth HS   – A late diastolic, presystolic sound is not heard in health and is a symptom of heart disease indicating resistance to ventricular filling (e.g.

The cadence caused by the addition of a third or fourth HS to the normal heart sounds is called a gallop rhythm.

Example

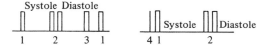

An opening snap (OS) occurring soon after the second HS is heard in mitral stenosis.

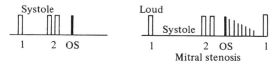

3. **Pericardial friction rub.** A to-and-fro superficial grating sound, usually heard in systole and diastole and often modified by posture. It suggests pericarditis.

4. **Murmurs.** Murmurs are less superficial and grating than friction rubs and may be systolic or diastolic in timing. It is important to remember that a murmur originating from a particular valve does not necessarily indicate disease of that valve. Increased blood flow, whether due to hyperdynamic circulation or to shunts between the right and left sides of the heart, may also give rise to murmurs from the valves through which the increased blood flow passes.

Listen in the following areas:

'Mitral': at apex
'Tricuspid': to left of lower end of sternum
'Aortic': to left of sternum in 2nd intercostal space
'Pulmonary': to left of sternum in 2nd intercostal space

Identification of murmurs

While listening you should note the following characteristics of a murmur:

Timing
Character
(*continued overleaf*)

27

Pitch

Intensity

Location (maximum intensity), e.g. apical, mitral, aortic or radiating up left sternal edge (ejection)

Extent and direction of transmission

Influence of respiration

1. Find where the murmur is loudest and then determine its **timing and character**

Pansystolic murmur

> – Mitral or tricuspid regurgitation; ventricular septal defect (VSD)

Ejection systolic murmur

> – Aortic or pulmonary stenosis; VSD or ASD; hyperdynamic circulation or normal

Early diastolic murmur

> – Aortic or pulmonary regurgitation

Mid-diastolic murmur

> – Mitral or tricuspid stenosis or large ASD

Continuous murmur

> – Patent ductus arteriosus (PDA)

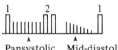

Pansystolic murmur   Mid-diastolic murmur

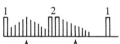

Ejection systolic murmur   Early diastolic murmur

2. What is the site of **maximum intensity and radiation** of the murmur?

> *In general* the murmur of:

> **Mitral regurgitation** is loudest at the apex and radiates to the axilla

> **Mitral stenosis** is located just internal to the apex

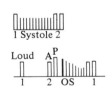

> **Tricuspid regurgitation or stenosis** is loudest over the lower sternum

> **Aortic stenosis** is loudest in the 2nd right intercostal space and radiates up into the carotids

28

Aortic regurgitation is loudest in
the 3rd and 4th left intercostal
spaces

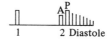

1   2 Diastole

**Pulmonary stenosis or regurgi-
tation** is loudest in the 2nd and
3rd left intercostal spaces

A VSD is loudest just to the left of the lower sternum

An ASD is a tricuspid and pulmonary flow murmur
(increased blood flow)

Systolic murmurs
Aortic stenosis/sclerosis
Mitral incompetence

Diastolic murmurs
Aortic incompetence (best heard with diaphragm of
stethoscope)
Mitral incompetence (best heard with bell of stethoscope)

3. Is it **louder on inspiration or expiration**? In general mitral and
aortic murmurs are loudest on expiration and pulmonary and
tricuspid murmurs on inspiration. Aortic murmurs are usually
best heard with the patient sitting forward and mitral murmurs
with the patient lying on the left side (after exercise if fit enough).

4. Does it have the **anticipated accompanying changes** in arterial
pulse, venous pulse, precordial impulses and heart sounds?

5. Is it an **insignificant** murmur? The decision that a murmur is
'innocent' is based upon the exclusion of organic causes. Insignificant murmurs are always systolic in timing and usually best heard
at the apex. By definition they have no associated features.

Minimal statement of the cardiovascular system (CVS)

(when no morbid signs exist)

Pulse 80/min; regular
BP 120/80 in right arm lying (•≪)
JVP not raised (often written: JVP – 0 or ↓)
No oedema (often written: oedema – 0)
Apex beat 5th intercostal space, 9 cm from midline
No evidence of right or left ventricular enlargement (often
written: RV – 0, LV – 0)
Heart sounds normal, no murmurs

or

Murmurs – 0

1   2

29

Examination of the respiratory system

The presence or absence of shortness of breath, cyanosis, clubbing and cough will already have been noted during the general examination and if not should always be ascertained in an examination of the respiratory system.

If the patient is **short of breath** note respiratory rate, depth, regularity, the use of accessory muscles (sterno-mastoids and scalenae), stridor and prolonged expiratory wheeze. In addition, at the end of the examination, measure peak flow rate (using a peak flow meter), forced expiratory volume in 1 minute (FEV_1) and forced vital capacity (FVC).

If the patient has a **productive cough** examine the sputum:

Mucoid suggests acute or chronic bronchitis

White or pink frothy suggests pulmonary oedema

Yellow or green suggests bacterial infection or eosinophilic sputum in asthma

Rusty coloured suggests pneumococcal pneumonia

Blood-stained suggests tumour, pulmonary embolus, TB or bronchiectasis

---

Examination of the chest

The front of the chest should be examined first (with the patient lying at 45°) and then the back (with the patient sitting upright). Avoid flitting from front to back.

Inspection

1. Note the **shape** of the chest, its symmetry and any spinal curvature.

    Exaggerated latero-posterior curvature of spine = kyphosis

    Lateral curvature of spine = scoliosis

    Barrel-shaped chest suggests obstructive airways disease

    Is the sternum depressed (pectus excavatum) or protuberant (pectus carinatum)?

2. Note the symmetry and extent of the **movements of the chest** on deep inspiration. In the absence of spinal deformity, diminished movement on one side usually indicates disease on that side. (*If in doubt* about the adequacy of chest move-

ments, measure the inspiratory to expiratory difference of chest circumference at nipple level – normally > 5 cm.)
3. Note any **inspiratory indrawing of the intercostal spaces**. (If pronounced, suggests airways obstruction.)
4. Note abnormal dilated veins on chest wall and operation scars.

Palpation

1. Check that the **trachea is central** by noting the position of the trachea relative to the tip of a finger placed in the suprasternal notch (the trachea may be displaced by tumours in the neck or upper mediastinum or by a shift of the mediastinum caused by lung collapse, massive pleural effusion or pneumothorax).
2. Confirm the findings on inspection:
   (*a*) the movements of the two sides of the chest;
   (*b*) the position of the apex beat
      (e.g. mediastinal displacement if the heart size is normal).
3. Compare the tactile vocal fremitus (TVF) on the two sides at two or three levels by placing the hand lightly on the chest, and asking the patient to repeat a resonant word (e.g. ninety-nine). It is usually *increased* over consolidated lung and *diminished* when air, fluid or a thickened pleura separates lung from chest wall, or when a major bronchus is obstructed.
4. If the complaint is of superficial chest pain, note any local rib tenderness (e.g. rib fracture, tumour or underlying pleurisy).

Percussion

Percuss the chest at several levels (four or five), comparing one side with the other (including the clavicles), and note the lower limits of pulmonary resonance on each side. This is much easier on the right side, where lung resonance gives way to liver dullness, than on the left where the lung resonance gives way to tympany of the stomach and large bowel. The note elicited on percussion (PN) is determined by the thickness of the chest wall, by the aeration of the lungs and by any structures intervening between the lung and the chest wall.

   Over normal lung, it is resonant
   Over liquid or solid, it is dull
   Over gas, under tension, it is tympanitic

Since the thickness of the chest wall varies from one subject to
another, the pitch of the note elicited is variable.

Auscultatory percussion

Auscultatory percussion involves gentle percussion over sternum
with simultaneous auscultation of lung fields over the back of the
chest; when increased this may indicate small areas of consolidation.

Examples

Dull percussion note

> – Over consolidated lung
> – Over a pleural effusion ('stony dull')
> – Over a large tumour
> – Over pleural thickening

Hyper-resonance

> – Over a pneumothorax
> – In patients with obstructive airways disease
>   (cause is lung hyperinflation, i.e. emphysema)
>   (cardiac and hepatic dullness may be lost)

Auscultation

Breath sounds (BS)

1. *Vesicular breath sounds.* Compare the breath sounds on
the two sides of the chest at three or four levels using either the
bell or the diaphragm. The noise generated by air passing through
the large airways during breathing is modified by conduction
through the normal lung and chest wall; thus the sound heard over
the thorax is softer and less harsh than that heard over the larynx.
In health, the inspiratory noise is clearly heard throughout inspiration whereas the expiratory noise is quieter, less harsh and usually only heard for the first half or two thirds of expiration. Such
normal sounds are called vesicular breath sounds.

2. *Diminished breath sounds.* The breath sounds are
diminished when thickened pleura, air or fluid separates the lung
from the chest wall and in thick-set muscular or obese individuals.
They are also diminished when the respiratory flow rate is con-
siderably reduced (e.g. severe asthma) and occasionally when the
relevant major bronchus is obstructed.
Do *not* describe diminished breath sounds as 'diminished air
entry' as this is not necessarily true.

3. *Bronchial breathing.* When the sound heard over the
thorax is similar to the sound heard over the larynx, i.e. is

unmodified by passage through aerated lung, the breath sounds are called bronchial breath sounds. These are heard over consolidated lung and at the upper level of a pleural effusion. Aegophony (a bleating sound on talking) and whispering pectoriloquy (harsh, easily heard whispered sounds) are inseparable auscultatory signs.

Added sounds (adventitious sounds)
Crackling sounds (râles), musical sounds (wheezes) and the sound caused by the two layers of the pleura rubbing together (pleural rub) may be heard. There is confusion about the origin and terminology of these sounds:

Old terminology		*New terminology*	
Râles	fine = crepitations medium coarse	= Crackles	fine medium coarse
Rhonchi	high-pitched = sibilant low-pitched = sonorous	= Wheezes	high-pitched low-pitched
Pleural rub		= Pleural rub	

It is no longer felt that fine, medium and coarse crackles are caused by air bubbling through fluid in fine-, medium- and wide-bore airways respectively. The sound is largely derived from the opening and closing of airways and does not necessarily imply intraluminal fluid. Similarly, the pitch of a wheeze does not indicate its origin, most being generated in large- and medium-sized airways. As the airways are normally narrower during expiration, wheezes are particularly pronounced during this phase.

Fine crackles (fine râles, crepitations) may be heard in pulmonary oedema, fibrosing alveolitis and during the early stages of pneumonic consolidation.

Medium and coarse crackles (medium and coarse râles) are characteristically associated with bronchiectasis and pneumonia but may be heard in severe pulmonary oedema, at the lung bases in emphysema and over bronchi containing secretions.

Wheezes (rhonchi) imply airways narrowing and are usually multiple and of varying pitch. A solitary localised wheeze, not abolished by coughing, indicates a localised airway narrowing and suggests a tumour, foreign body or inspissated mucus.

Pleural rubs indicate pleural inflammation but do not differentiate between inflammation caused by infection, neoplasia, autoimmune disease or ischaemia/infarction.

(when no morbid signs exist)

> No cyanosis, clubbing
> No lymphadenopathy
> Respiratory rate 16/min
> No shortness of breath
> Shape normal
> Movements normal
> Trachea central
> Percussion note resonant all areas
>   PN of right = PN of left = normal
> Breath sounds vesicular, no added sounds

Signs useful in differentiating between respiratory conditions

Condition	Tactile fremitus	Percussion note	Breath sounds
Obstructive airways disease (asthma, emphysema)	Normal or decreased	Normal or increased	Prolonged expiration ± wheeze
Pneumonic consolidation	Normal or increased	Decreased	Bronchial breathing ± crackles
Pleural effusion	Decreased	Decreased	Decreased
Pneumothorax	Decreased	Normal or increased	Decreased
Pulmonary oedema	Normal	Normal	Fine crackles

Examination of the alimentary system

The presence or absence of anaemia, jaundice, peripheral stigmata or cirrhosis such as spider naevi, palmar erythema and gynaecomastia, signs of iron deficiency such as koilonychia and smooth tongue, and skin rashes associated with certain gastro-intestinal conditions will already have been noted during the general examination.

Examination of the oro-pharynx

Examine lips, gums, teeth, tongue, tonsils and palate.

Soreness at corners of the mouth (angular cheilosis)
- Suggests iron or riboflavin (vitamin B_2) deficiency or ill-fitting dentures

Tongue – Dry or moist

Smooth atrophic tongue
- Suggests iron or vitamin B_{12} deficiency

Aphthous ulceration
- More commonly suggests local trauma or infection; may indicate coeliac or inflammatory bowel disease

Dark pigmentation inside the cheeks (buccal pigmentation)
- Suggests hypoadrenalism

Teeth – Natural or false

Dental caries – Important in management of rheumatic valve disease

Spongy bleeding gums
- More commonly suggests poor dental hygiene; may indicate leukaemia

Hypertrophied gums
- Side-effect of phenytoin (an anticonvulsant)

Examination of the abdomen

Examine the abdomen in good light with the patient lying flat with arms by the side. Cross light is better than full illumination. The patient's confidence must be gained if a satisfactory examination is to be made, and warm hands go a long way to securing this.

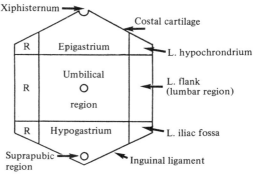

Always note:

Abnormal distension
 – General or local
Operation scars – Are they anticipated from the history?
Visible peristalsis
 – Unless the patient is very thin this suggests intestinal obstruction
Protuberant umbilicus
 – Suggests umbilical hernia or ascites
Distended veins and direction of flow
 – May indicate portal hypertension or obstruction of the inferior vena cava

Palpation

1. **Palpate each quadrant** and note areas of **tenderness** or **guarding** (a resistance to palpation due to voluntary contraction of the abdominal wall muscles). If appendicitis is suspected, palpate **McBurney's point** (one third of the way along a line drawn from the right anterior superior iliac spine to the umbilicus). To determine whether mild degrees of tenderness or guarding indicate peritoneal inflammation, press the fingers into the tender area as far as possible and then suddenly remove them. If removing the fingers in this way gives rise to pain (**rebound tenderness**), peritoneal inflammation is suggested.
2. Localised or generalised **rigidity** of the abdominal wall muscles suggests local or generalised peritonitis. When severe it is termed board-like rigidity.
3. **Palpate the liver** by placing the hand flat on the abdomen with the straight edge of the index finger parallel to and just below the right costal margin in the nipple line. The hand is then depressed slightly as the patient takes a deep breath and the diaphragm brings the liver to it. If palpable, describe its size (by also percussing the upper margin in the right chest, between the anterior and mid-axillary lines), its position, consistency and the condition of the surface and edge. (If impalpable, start again in right iliac fossa.)

   The **gallbladder** is not palpable unless enlarged and even then is only palpable with difficulty. Inflammation of the gallbladder may be detected by pressing the fingers into the right hypochondrium as the patient takes a deep breath.

Sudden pain when the gallbladder touches the fingers indicates inflammation (**Murphy's sign**), as also does hyper-
aesthesia over thoracic segments 9, 10 and 11 posteriorly on
the right side (**Boas' sign**).
4. **Palpate for the spleen**, and if palpable note its size. If
splenomegaly is anticipated but not detected in the supine
position, palpate bimanually with the patient lying on the
right side and the left arm in a relaxed position over the side
of the chest wall so the left hand just touches the right
shoulder.
5. **Palpate for the kidneys**, and if palpable (rare in healthy subjects unless thin) describe their position, size, consistency,
shape and mobility with respiration. Bimanual palpation
with one hand in the flank posteriorly and one hand
anteriorly may be necessary. Distinguishing signs between
enlarged left kidney and enlarged spleen are:
  Left kidney mass is bimanually palpable, spleen is not
  Fingers can usually reach above upper pole of kidney,
    not so for spleen
  Spleen has a notch on its inferior margin, kidney does
    not
  Spleen enlarges towards right iliac fossa, left kidney
    towards left iliac fossa
  Area of resonance to percussion over kidney but not
    spleen
  Area of dullness over Traub's space in enlarged spleen
6. Can any **tumour** be felt in the abdomen? If it can, describe
its position (especially in respect of its relation to other
organs), size, consistency, shape, and mobility.
7. Is there any **gastric splash** to be elicited? (This suggests
pyloric obstruction.)
8. Inspect and palpate the **hernial orifices**; this is often facili-
tated by asking the patient to cough.
Direct inguinal hernia usually bulges forward above the
inguinal ligament.
Indirect inguinal hernia passes through the internal inguinal
ring along the inguinal canal, emerging through the
external inguinal ring (above and medial to the pubic
tubercle) and into the scrotum or labia majora.
Femoral hernia emerges from the femoral canal which lies
below and lateral to the pubic tubercle.
When a hernia is present, note whether coughing produces
a palpable impulse (excludes strangulation) and whether it
is tender and reducible.

This is used to identify the presence of free or encysted fluid in the abdomen and to determine whether palpable tumours are superficial or deep. It may help to determine the size of the liver and spleen if abdominal rigidity prevents adequate palpation.

Shifting dullness is a sign of free fluid in the peritoneal cavity (e.g. cirrhotic ascites). With the patient lying on his/her back percuss the areas of dullness, which in the presence of fluid are in the dependent parts of the abdomen. Mark the limits of resonance in the umbilical plane on the left side and then turn the patient on to the right side and again mark the limits of resonance. Sometimes in a normal subject the limits of resonance may move through 3–5 cm as the gaseous and liquid contents of the gut move, but with free fluid this movement is usually much greater.

The smaller amount of an ascites can be detected by putting the patient in the knee–elbow position and percussing the abdomen from beneath. The fluid will collect around the umbilicus and give rise to an area of dullness there.

When the abdomen is distended with fluid, a **fluid thrill** may be elicited. This may be determined by a firm tap on one flank detected by the other hand placed on the opposite flank, with an observer's hand placed lengthwise (along the side of the hand and little finger) along the centre of the abdomen over the umbilicus.

Auscultation

The chief use of auscultation is to determine the frequency and intensity of bowel sounds (borborygmi). Listen in the four quadrants of the abdomen and note the interval between intestinal sounds and their pitch.

In **intestinal obstruction**, the sounds are often more frequent, louder, high-pitched and tinkling.

In **paralytic ileus**, which may accompany generalised peritonitis, the sounds are absent.

Friction rubs may be audible over splenic or hepatic infarcts or tumours as the patient breathes. Note arterial murmurs or venous hums (can be heard over tumours particularly in the liver).

38

Examination of the rectum

This should be performed in all patients, but may be deferred, unless relevant, if the patient is very ill. It is suggested that you do this at the same time as the House Officer, to avoid unnecessary discomfort and embarrassment for the patient.

1. Place the patient in a curled up position lying on the left side.
2. Examine the anus, noting whether there are any external haemorrhoids, fissures or other abnormalities.
3. After inserting a gloved forefinger (usually the right) covered with lubricating jelly, note the condition of the anal sphincter and the presence or absence of faeces in the rectum.
   In a male patient palpate the prostate and describe its size and consistency and whether or not the median groove is palpable.
4. If a tumour is felt, note its size, situation, consistency, shape and mobility.
5. Can pain be produced by pressure in any part of the rectum and if so in which direction?
6. Describe any other abnormality which can be felt.
7. Did examination cause bleeding?

Minimal statement of the alimentary system (AS)

(when no morbid signs exist)

Mouth – mucosa, fauces and teeth normal
Abdomen – soft, no tenderness or rigidity
Normal bowel sounds
Liver, spleen, kidneys and bladder not palpable
No abnormal masses felt   *or*:
Hernial orifices normal
Rectal examination (PR)
  – normal

L = 0   S = 0

K = 0   o   K = 0

39

Examination of the external genitalia

Male

(chaperoned in the case of female students)

> Note distribution of **pubic hair** (male escutcheon).
> Note any obvious abnormalities of the **penis** (e.g. small size, penile discharge, hypospadias, phimosis (tight prepuce covering the glans) or paraphimosis (tight prepuce surrounding the base of the glans)).
> Examine the **scrotum** and both **testes** (if absent seek along their line of descent).
> Note testicular size (normal adult 3–5 cm in length), consistency (usually firm, but small and soft in cirrhosis and hypogonadism).
> Note any swellings such as a testicular tumour (often impalpable), a **spermatocoele** (a retention cyst of the vasa efferentia lying above and behind the testis), a **hydrocoele** (accumulation of fluid within the tunica vaginalis of the testis, which may almost surround the testis and which may be transilluminated when a torch is pressed against it), and a **varicocoele** (varicosity of testicular veins, evident when the patient is standing).

Female

(only to be done when appropriate and when chaperoned in the case of male students)

> Note distribution of **pubic hair**.
> Note obvious abnormalities of **introitus**.
> Note enlargement of **clitoris** (suggests androgen excess).
> Vaginal examination should only be done in the presence of the House officer and when appropriate.

Minimal statement of the genito-urinary system (GUS)

(when no morbid signs exist)

> External genitalia – normal

40

Examination of the nervous system

Obvious muscle weakness, involuntary movements and impairment of level of consciousness will already have been noted. The scheme given below is for a detailed examination, but a 'screening' examination of the cranial nerves, limb power and reflexes will suffice when neurological disease is not anticipated (see Minimal statement of the nervous system, p. 52).

Assessment of higher cerebral function

Formal assessment of higher cerebral function is usually unnecessary if an articulate history and a co-operative examination can be given by the patient.

(i) *Attention* (conscious level)

Impaired consciousness varies from mild drowsiness to deep coma. Describe its degree and pattern of response to certain stimuli such as spoken voice and painful pressure (e.g. squeeze of ear lobe).

Examples

Drowsy but moves all limbs to command

Unconscious and no response to command but moves left limbs in response to painful stimuli

If conscious level is impaired, further tests of higher cerebral function are usually irrelevant. (Impaired consciousness may have a metabolic or neurological cause.)

If conscious level is normal, test:

Orientation in time and place by asking the *date* and *place*. Patients with diffuse cerebral lesions, drug intoxication and certain metabolic disorders may be disorientated but alert. (This test has little localising value.)

Attentiveness of patient by *digit span test* (normal: six or seven figures).

(ii) *Cognitive skills* (learned mental activities)

The basic cognitive skills are the ability to speak, understand speech, read, write and perceive objects. These skills are related

to the left hemisphere in 99% of right-handed subjects and 60– **41**
70% of left-handed subjects and are functions of the parietal and
temporal regions. Assessment of these skills may have considerable localising value but of course the educational background of
the subject must be taken into account when these functions are
examined. The importance of establishing dominance is obvious.

Dysphasia is impairment in understanding or expressing language
(usually a lesion of the dominant hemisphere). In testing speech
function distinction must be made between dysphasia (see above)
and dysarthria, which is a disorder of articulation due to a paresis
or incoordination of the peripheral mechanism for speech production (e.g. larynx, tongue or lips).

> *Expressive dysphasia*: inability to express by the spoken
> word. Ask the patient the meaning of a simple proverb.
> (Inability suggests tempoparietal lesion.)
> *Receptive dysphasia*: failure to understand the spoken word
> or a command. Ask the patient to touch the left ear with
> the right hand. (Impairment suggests posterior parietal
> lesion.)
> *Nominal dysphasia*: inability to name objects (e.g. parts of a
> watch). (Inability suggests temporal lobe lesion.)

Dyscalculia is impairment in calculation. Ask the patient to
serially subtract 7 from 100. (Impairment suggests parietal
lesion.)

Constructional apraxia is the inability to orientate in space. Ask
the patient to copy a five-pointed star. (Impairment suggests posterior parietal lesion or metabolic derangement.)

Other tests suggesting a parietal lesion include:

> **Unilateral neglect**: suggests sensory inattention (see tests of
> sensory function).
> **Apraxia**: disturbance in ability to perform a purposeful act
> when comprehension is intact (given a fork, the patient
> may be unable to use it to eat).
> **Dyslexia**: impairment in reading.
> **Dysgraphia**: impairment in writing.

(iii) *Memory*

Memory loss may vary and also can be useful in localising a lesion.

> *Short-term memory*: ask the patient to repeat a series of
> five, six or seven numbers in correct order, the normal

digit span being six or seven figures. (Impairment suggests parietal lesion.)

Verbal memory: test with a name and address or with recent current events, a short story of the 'Babcock sentence' ('The one thing a nation needs in order to be rich and great, is a large, secure supply of wood'). Most subjects can repeat this after one or two hearings. (Impairment suggests temporal lesion.)

Visual memory: recognition of photographs of well-known personalities. (Impairment suggests right temporal lesion.)

(iv) *Reason and problem-solving*

Subtle impairment of these parameters may occur in the absence of other derangement but may be difficult to demonstrate as bedside tests are insensitive and the patient's attempts are influenced by IQ. Test reason and problem-solving by asking the patient to repeat four digits in reverse order or by asking how many 6p oranges can be bought for 40p. (Impairment suggests widespread cerebral disease or frontal lesion.)

Examination of skull, neck and cranial nerves

Skull and neck

Note shape of skull and listen over skull, orbits and neck for bruits (e.g. with carotid stenosis, arterio-venous malformation).

Check for neck stiffness (suggests meningitis or subarachnoid haemorrhage).

Kernig's sign (inability to extend lower leg when that leg is flexed at the hip) is also a test of meningeal irritation.

Cranial nerves

I: Smell. Only tested when frontal tumour or fracture suspected.

Rough test: smell flowers (subjectively)

Formal test: smelling bottles

It is the appreciation of smell by each nostril and not identification of smell that is important. (Commonest cause of impairment is nasal mucosa inflammation.)

II: Visual acuity. Allow patient to wear glasses if worn.

Rough test: reading

Snellen chart (distant vision)

If acuity is severely impaired note ability to count fingers, observe hand movements, perceive or not perceive light. (Refractive errors of the lens are the commonest cause of visual impairment.)

Colour vision

(lost early in optic neuritis)

> Rough test: equal appreciation of coloured object (red) by each eye
>
> Formal test: Ischihara chart

Fields of vision

Rough test of peripheral fields (by confrontation): Examiner and patient sit approximately 1 metre apart facing each other. Each covers one opposing eye and stares into the opposite open eye of the other person (e.g. examiner right and patient left eye). The examiner then brings his/her hand (or the head of a hat pin) from the periphery into his/her own field of vision midway between himself/herself and the patient from positions right, left, above and below and confirms that the patient sees the object at the same time as he/she does himself/herself. The test is repeated with the opposite eye.

> Formal testing of peripheral and central fields: Bjerrum screen.

> Defects in the visual fields (hemianopia) are of considerable localising value if the anatomy of the optic pathways is known.

Fundus oculi with ophthalmoscope.

Note:

> Opacities in the cornea, anterior chamber, lens and vitreous humour
>
> Size, colour and contour of the optic disc
>
> Distribution and size of retinal arteries and veins
>
> Presence of exudates, haemorrhages and pigment

III, IV, VI: Supply the **external ocular muscles** (EOM): (VI lateral rectus, IV superior oblique and III the rest). In addition, III supplies the levator palpebrae superioris and carries parasympathetic fibres to the muscles of accommodation and the sphincter pupillae (constrictor). The afferent limb of the light reflex is conveyed in the optic nerve (II). Sympathetic dilator fibres to the sphincter pupillae arise in the cervical sympathetic chain and are conveyed to the eye with the internal carotid artery and thence the ophthalmic division of V.

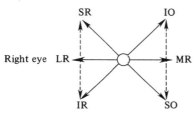

Key

IR   Inferior rectus
LR   Lateral rectus
MR Medial rectus
SR   Superior rectus
IO   Inferior oblique
SO   Superior oblique

(Direction of EOM action in abducted or adducted positions is shown in broken lines.)

Examples

1. III paresis: eye points down and outwards (because of over-action of LR + SO)

2. IV paresis: eye cannot look down and in

3. VI paresis: eye cannot look laterally

When assessing functioning of the III, IV and VI nerves:

Examine eyelids for ptosis (suggests III nerve or sympathetic lesion).

Examine pupils for size. shape, reaction to light (direct and consensual) and accommodation.

Partial ptosis and ipsilateral small pupil suggest cervical sympathetic lesion (Horner's syndrome).

Irregularly shaped small pupil that reacts to accommodation but not to light suggests neurosyphilis (Argyll–Robertson pupil), diabetes.

Look for squint (strabismus) on forward gaze. If both eyes can be shown to have full movements when tested individually with the other eye closed, the squint is likely to be of long standing (concomitant with squint of childhood).

Test eye movements laterally to the right and left, up and down, noting squint or complaint of double vision.

Test for nystagmus (jerky eye movements). Test laterally

and upwards but remain within the limits of binocular
vision. Symmetrical nystagmus outside fields of
binocular vision need not be pathological. Nystagmus
may result from retinal, vestibular or cerebellar lesions
and sometimes from drug intoxication (e.g. barbitu-
rates).

V: Supplies **sensory fibres to face and cornea** (V^1, V^2, V^3) and
motor fibres to jaw.
Test:

> Sensation on face to light touch and pin-prick
> Corneal reflex (involuntary blink when unseen wisp of wool
> touches cornea from the side)
> Bulk of masseter and temporal muscles when jaw is
> clenched
> Integrity of pterygoids by opening jaw against resistance
> Jaw jerk

VII: Facial symmetry. Assess both upper (screwing up eyes) and
lower (showing teeth) parts of the face, as upper part of the face
is bilaterally represented in the cortex. Hence unilateral weakness
of the lower part of the face suggests **upper motor neurone lesion**
(UMN), whereas complete unilateral weakness suggests **lower
motor neurone lesion** (LMN) (Bell's palsy).

VIII: Auditory hearing. Confirm that the patient can hear the
sound of fingers rubbed together close to the ear *or* the ticking of
a watch *or* whispered words. If hearing is impaired, compare air
and bone conduction with a tuning fork (**Rinne's test**). Air conduction is normally better than bone conduction (AC > BC).
Also note ear in which sound is heard when a tuning fork is placed
on the forehead (**Weber's test**).

Vestibular. Vestibular nerve is connected with the cerebellum.
Abnormalities of the nerve may be associated with nystagmus,
vertigo and ataxia.

> Look for *nystagmus*, which is a disturbance of ocular pos-
> ture characterised by involuntary rhythmical oscillation
> of the eyes. The movements can be horizontal, vertical or
> rotary. To examine for nystagmus, ask the patient to look
> straight in front of him and observe whether the eyes
> remain steady. Then ask him to look to the right and to
> the left. Observe the flickering movement in each direc-
> tion, the quicker component of the movement indicates
> the direction of the nystagmus. Nystagmus can also be
> due to visual disorders, weakness of ocular muscles and
> cerebellar disorders.

46

Vertigo will be decribed by the patient as giddiness or dizziness. In true vertigo, objects appear to move around the patient.

Ataxia or incoordination. may be tested by asking the patient to stand erect with eyes open and noting a tendency to fall backwards or more rarely fall forwards. Ataxia is also associated with cerebellar disorders.

IX, X: Note asymmetry of palate on saying 'aah'. If impairment anticipated or deviation of palate noted above, test 'gag reflex' by touching posterior pharyngeal wall with orange stick. (Patient may also demonstrate nasal regurgitation on swallowing, dysarthria (see p. 41), dysphagia and a bovine cough).

XI: Test trapezius (shrugging shoulders) and sterno-mastoid (lifting head from pillow against resistance).

XII: Note deviation of tongue on protrusion, wasting and fasciculation ('bag of worms').

Examination of motor functions of the limbs and trunk

When neurological disease is not anticipated examination of the motor functions of the limbs is usually limited to excluding muscle wasting, and testing muscle tone and power around the major joints and the major reflexes (see Minimal statement of the nervous system, p. 52).

Tone

This may be:

> Normal
>
> Decreased, as in lower motor neurone and cerebellar lesions
>
> Increased, as in upper motor neurone lesions ('clasp knife rigidity' and 'clonus') or in extrapyramidal lesions ('cogwheel rigidity')

Muscle weakness or paralysis

This may be due to:

> Myopathy or neuromuscular block (e.g. myasthaenia gravis)
>
> Lower motor neurone lesion: muscles wasted, flaccid with fasciculation ('bag of worms' appearance due to

unstimulated flickering of fibres) and reflexes absent; plantar response flexor or absent

Upper motor neurone lesion (pyramidal): muscles not wasted, spastic (clasp knife type) and exaggerated reflexes; plantar response extensor. Weakness least and tone greatest in flexors of arm and extensors of leg

The degree of muscle weakness may be recorded as follows:

0   No contraction
1   Flicker or trace of contraction
2   Active movement with gravity eliminated
3   Active movement against gravity
4   Active movement against gravity and resistance
5   Normal power

Examination of the upper limbs

Look for wasting, fasciculation and involuntary movements

Assess tone at wrist and elbow

Test power of

Flexors of fingers – Grip hands
Extensors of fingers – Extension of outstretched fingers
Dorsal interossei (T1) – Finger abduction
Abductor pollicis brevis – Abduction of thumb
Flexors and extensors (C8) of wrist
Flexors (C6) and extensors (C7) of elbow
Deltoid (C5) – Shoulder abduction

Assess coordination

Ask patient to touch repeatedly first his/her nose and then your finger placed approximately 60 cm away, using first one forefinger and then the other (the finger–nose test).

If he/she succeeds without faltering no incoordination is present. The coordination of movements is governed particularly by the cerebellum. It cannot be satisfactorily assessed in the presence of muscle weakness or loss of position sense.

Note grade of reflex:

Normal   +
Reduced   ±
Increased   + +
Absent   —

Muscle	Root base	Right	Left
Biceps	C5, 6	+	+
Triceps	C6, 7	+	+
Supinator	C5, 6	+	+
Finger flexion	C7, 8	+	+

If tendon reflexes are absent, test again with reinforcement (= Jendrassik's manoeuvre: isometric contraction on the hands against each other).

Examination of the lower limbs

Look for wasting, fasciculation and involuntary movements

Assess tone at hip, knee and ankle (clonus)

Test power of

> Extensors (L4, 5) and flexors (S1) of ankle
> Invertors and evertors (L5) of ankle
> Extensors (L3, 4) and flexors of knee
> Extensors and flexors (L2, 3) of hip
> Abductors and adductors of hip

Assess coordination

1. Ask the patient to rub heel down opposite shin
2. Ask the patient to walk along a straight line
3. Observe gait

Test reflexes

Note grade of reflex as for upper limbs

Reflex	Root base	Right	Left
Knee	L3, 4	+	+
Ankle	S1, 2	+	+
Plantars		↓	↓

Examination of the trunk

Test power of

Extensors and flexors of the head
Abdominal muscles

Abdominal reflexes

Note grade of reflex as for upper limbs. Record upper and lower
abdominal reflexes as shown:

Right	Left
+	+
+	+

Examination of sensory functions of the limbs and trunk

Sensory functions of the limbs and trunk are often difficult
to test and are therefore assessed only when indicated. The indi-
cation may be obvious, e.g. when the subject has sensory
symptoms or has a laceration that may have damaged a sensory
nerve. Sometimes, however, the sensory system is examined to
seek an abnormality of which the patient is unaware, e.g. a
peripheral neuropathy in a diabetic patient.

For the assessment to be meaningful, it is vital that the
patient is relaxed, that the examination is not prolonged, that the
patient does not see the various stimuli administered and that he
is a good sensory witness. Owing to the large number of different
sensory end-organs, examination is limited to those stimuli most
likely to demonstrate an abnormality at the level of the nervous
system under suspicion. Thus:

Peripheral nerve

Light touch (cotton wool)
Superficial pain (pin-prick)
Establish dermatome involved (see figure p. 51)

Superficial pain	Contralateral anterior
Deep pain (squeezing muscles)	and lateral spino-
Temperature (hot and cold)	thalamic tract
Vibration sense	Ipsilateral posterior
Position sense in	columns
fingers and toes	

Romberg's test: If the patient is able to stand up straight with the eyes open, but stumbles when the eyes are closed, he/she has probably lost position sense in the lower limbs.

Cerebral cortex (parietal lesions)

Two-point discrimination

Ability to recognise shape, size and form of objects placed in the hand (**stereognosis**)

Sensory inattention. Lesions above the thalamus do not abolish the appreciation of sensation but may raise the threshold. Thus in a patient with a **parietal lesion** the sensations evoked by touching each limb individually may appear similar. However, when the limbs are touched simultaneously the stimulus from the contra-lateral side to the parietal lesion may not be appreciated (i.e. unilateral neglect). This may also be noted when testing visual fields.

Hysterical sensory loss tends to correspond to a part of the body (e.g. arm, hand or midline of the trunk) rather than the actual innervation of the skin and can be altered by suggestion. One way of testing it is to place a vibrating tuning fork on each side of the sternum in turn. Appreciation of the vibrating sensation depends on bone conduction and not superficial sensory pathways limited to dermatomes and thus one should be suspicious if the patient claims that the sensation is different on the two sides. This test may also be used to determine whether the patient is a good sensory witness.

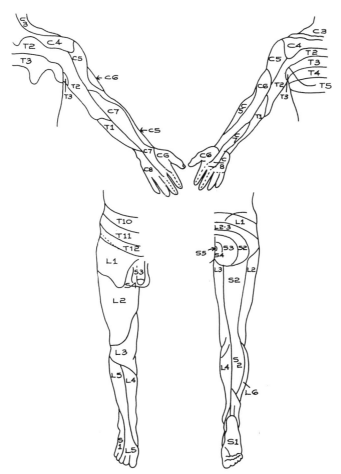

52

Examination of the autonomic nervous system

The autonomic nervous system is not examined routinely but symptoms such as postural hypotension, diarrhoea, impotence and loss of sweating for which no other cause can be found, may suggest an autonomic neuropathy (e.g. diabetes mellitus).

Parasympathetic

Test **afferent** arc by confirming:

Increase in heart rate on standing
Normal blood pressure 'overshoot' and bradycardia after Valsalva manoeuvre

Test **efferent** arc by confirming increase of heart rate when vagus is blocked by atropine (only to be done under supervision).

Sympathetic

Test **afferent** arc by demonstrating sweat production in response to heat.
Test **efferent** arc by confirming:

Rise in blood pressure when noradrenaline is infused (only under supervision)
Piloerection with local injection of acetylcholine (only under supervision)

Minimal statement of the nervous system (CNS)

(when no morbid signs exist)

Alert and co-operative
Right handed. Skull and spine normal
Cranial nerves II–XII normal
Pupils equal, regular, react equally to light and accommodation (PERLA)
Optic fundi normal
Eye movements (EOM) not impaired. No nystagmus
Limbs – tone, power and coordination normal
Reflexes – all present and equal, plantars flexor
Sensation grossly normal

53

Examination of the locomotor system

Most observations for abnormality in this system will have been made during the examination of the nervous system. Muscle wasting, joint deformity, pain or crepitus should be noted.

Suggested scheme for examining joints

Always compare the abnormal joint with its counterpart in the opposite limb.

Inspection. Note swelling in and around the joint, redness, shiny appearance of the overlying skin and position in which the joint is held, as well as deformity.

Palpation. Note increased skin temperature, presence of fluid within joint or its bursa, swelling of synovial membrane and areas of tenderness.

Movement. Note crepitus (palpable grating sensation) and range of movement (limited or excessive). Note whether limited movement is caused by pain or by mechanical factors within or outside the joint. If an infective process is thought to be responsible, palpate regional lymph nodes.

Examination of the spine

In general this examination is best performed with the patient standing and dressed only in undergarments.

Inspection. Note kyphosis, scoliosis, lordosis (posterior curvature of the spine is normal in the lumbar region), asymmetry of spinal muscles and abnormal lumps.

Palpation. Gently palpate the spine. Local spinal tenderness suggests a lesion of the underlying vertebrae or adjacent structures.

Movement. Note the range of spinal movement in flexion, extension, lateral flexion and rotation. Also note postures giving rise to local or referred pain.

Special tests used for patients with low back pain

Note tenderness of the sacro-iliac joints.
With patient lying supine, flex the legs at the hip (one at a

time) keeping the knee extended and note the development of low back pain or pain referred to the buttock or to the posterolateral aspect of the leg (sciatica). This indicates pressure upon the sciatic nerve (L4, L5, S1) and is usually caused by posterolateral protrusion of an intervertebral disc. Sciatic pain is often brought on by coughing or sneezing (by raising cerebrospinal fluid pressure in the spinal subarachnoid space).

With patient lying prone, extend the legs at the hip and note the development of pain along the front of the thigh (femoral stretch test). This indicates pressure on the femoral nerve (L2, L3) and is usually caused by disc protrusion or osteoarthritis of the lumbar spine.

Also note muscle wasting, weakness, cutaneous sensory loss and abnormality of reflexes.

Examination of the limbs

The limbs should be examined as a whole first and then segment by segment, the two sides being compared.

Note valgus (away from midline) and varus (towards the midline): deformities of elbows, knees, ankles and feet.

Note abnormalities of the joints, their movements and associated muscle wasting.

Measurement of leg length

One leg may appear shorter than the other either because it is (true shortening) or because the hip is tilted (apparent shortening).

True shortening is demonstrated by measuring the distance between the anterior iliac spine and the medial malleolus of the two legs (the longer leg being placed in a similar position to the shorter leg).

Apparent shortening is demonstrated by measuring the distance between the xiphisternum and the medial malleolus on each side (with the legs parallel).

Gait

The patient should be asked to walk up and down, as this may demonstrate functional abnormality in the lower limbs and, less often, in the upper limbs.

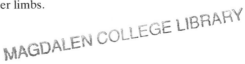

Minimal statement of the locomotor system
(when no morbid signs are present)

    Spine normal
    Joints normal
    Gait normal

56

Scheme for taking a psychiatric history

Complaints

Write down the patient's presenting complaints, verbatim if possible.

History of the present complaint

Obtain a detailed account of the illness from the earliest time a change was noted. The *sequence* of the various symptoms should be dated approximately, and a record made of changes in the patient's life situation as a result of the illness, and his* reaction to them (e.g. sick leave or loss of job, limitation of social activities, estrangement from spouse, conflict with the law). Note the reason for, and mode of, admission to hospital.

Do not limit yourself to a mere statement of the patient's spontaneous complaints. You should enquire about other important symptoms, especially presence or absence of other psychological symptoms.

For example, a complaint of 'depression' should always be followed by questions about the quality of the mood change and any variation, concentration, interest, energy, sleep, appetite, guilt, self-pity, etc.

Previous history

Psychiatric:	– Note any previous nervous or mental illness; whether or not in circumscribed attacks; whether treated and if so where
Medical:	– Covered previously

* For simplicity the female pronoun has not been used in this section, though it is intended throughout that 'the patient' could be either male or female.

57

Family history

Parents:	– Age, occupation and health. (If deceased, age at death and cause. Note patient's age at death of parent.) Personality
Sibs:	– List in chronological order (with Christian name) age, marital state, occupation, health, personality. Record the presence of any nervous or mental trouble, including heavy drinking
Early home environment:	– At this point it is convenient to enquire about the environment in which the patient spent his childhood (e.g. whether brought up by parents or others), home atmosphere, relations between parents and between parents and children. Financial state of family and material environment

Personal history

Date and place of birth:	– Full term or premature; normal delivery or otherwise; birth injuries
Health during childhood:	– Delicate or healthy; as mentioned previously
Neurotic traits:	– Excessive 'nervousness' or shyness; also enuresis, food fads, temper tantrums, sleep-walking
School record:	– School leaving age. Names and types of schools attended and academic progress; success in making friends; ability to relate to teacher; participation in games; home-sickness; disciplinary difficulties
Work record:	– List, in chronological order, jobs held, with reasons for taking and leaving them. Also note any service in the forces and rank
Sexual and marital adjustment:	
Marital:	– Age at marriage. Duration of acquaintance before marriage and of engagement. Spouse's age, occupation and personality. Compatibility; sharing of responsibilities. Sexual difficulties; contraceptive measures. List of

children with names and ages and brief note of
health and personality of each

Sex: – Age at onset of puberty (menarche, voice-
breaking) and how regarded. In female
patients, regularity of periods, and presence
of pain or emotional disturbance before or
during them; also age at menopause and any
accompanying physical or psychological
disturbance

The following topics are often embarrassing to patients and if not
immediately relevant may be omitted. However, if there is any
evidence of sexual difficulty or unusual sexual interest, these
areas will have to be explored:

– Knowledge of the facts of life and how
acquired. Masturbation, associated fantasies
and attitudes towards them. Sexual experi-
ences and attitudes towards them. Homo-
sexual feelings during adolescence or later

Present home – Attitude to housing; financial and social
situation: circumstances. Problems in family relation-
ships and recent stresses within and outside
the home

Personality before illness

The personal history may indicate stability, permanency,
ability to accept responsibility and whether the patient is positive
and effective, or negative and inadequate. Also how far the
present state contrasts with his previous personality.
Additional points to be enquired for are:

Social relations: – Attitudes towards relatives and friends, ability
to mix easily. Attitudes towards authority
(including anti-social trends, stealing, lying,
etc.), towards religion and politics. Record
any group activities in clubs, societies, etc.
How is leisure spent? Hobbies and interests.
Social aspirations

Mood: – Whether habitually cheerful or despondent.
Anxious or placid. Optimistic or pessimistic.
Warm-hearted or emotionally cold. Ask
particularly whether mood is relatively stable

	or prone to fluctuations, regular or irregular, and whether predictable or not
Character:	– Self-confident or shy and timid. Self-reliant in planning and judgement or dependent on others; enterprising or preferring the old familiar. Ask particularly whether patient is scrupulous, conscientious, prone to set himself high standards, punctual and methodical, or capricious, unreliable, impulsive. (Strictness, fussiness and rigid adherence to routine are often associated with extreme conscientiousness.)
Activity:	– Whether active and energetic or sluggish and easily fatigued. Whether energy output is sustained or fitful
Habits:	– Food fads; excretory function; alcohol; tobacco; drugs. Concern over health; frequent taking of patent medicines

Medical state at interview

Appearance and behaviour:	– Tidy or ill-kempt? Calm, tense or agitated? Cheerful or glum? Easy or difficult to make contact with? Any noticeable oddities such as mannerisms or gestures?
Mood:	– Appearance gives some indication of this. Non-committal questions should be asked: 'How do you feel in yourself?' 'How are your spirits?' Many varieties of mood may be present – not merely degrees of happiness or sadness, but irritability, fear, worry, bewilderment, apathy. Note how constant the mood is, whether the patient seems capable of 'snapping out of it' temporarily, and how far the mood is appropriate to the circumstances
Talk:	– Form rather than content is considered here. Does the patient talk readily or reluctantly? At normal speed or very fast or very slowly? To the point or discursively? Is the patient coherent? Any strange words or puns? Any sudden stops or changes of topic? **Give verbatim examples**

Thought content:	– (i) *Preoccupations and fears* – of ill-health, insanity, poverty, guilt, etc. Any obsessive–compulsive phenomena, i.e. thoughts or impulses repeatedly intruding against the patient's will? Does he have to repeat actions unnecessarily? Does he realise their illogicality?
	(ii) *Delusions and misinterpretations*: Does the patient show abnormal attitudes towards people or things? Is he treated well or in some special way by people around him? Are people talking about him or looking at him? Does he feel under any influence or control? Has he had perplexing experiences? Does he read in the papers, see on TV or hear on the radio, things referring specifically to him? Does he deprecate and blame himself (e.g. in his morals, character, health or possessions) or does he seem to regard himself in an inflated, grandiose way? **Give verbatim examples**
	(iii) *Disorders of perception*: Does he see things? Do his thoughts turn to words in his head? Does he hear voices giving him orders or criticising him or interfering with his thoughts? Does he experience peculiar bodily sensations, vibrations or electricity etc.? Note the frequency, vividness and timing of hallucinations, as well as the patient's reaction to them and beliefs about their origin. **Give verbatim examples**
Intellectual functions:	– Assessed as in section on neurological examination (pp. 40–2).

Physical examination

As suggested earlier in the booklet.

61

Documentation of the medical record

The history and examination

These should be recorded as already described. In addition you should:

> Summarise the history and examination (positive findings)
> Construct a provisional or differential diagnosis
> Enumerate investigations required
> Decide upon a course of management
> Write up progress notes (and operation notes)
> Write your own discharge note

Summary of positive findings

This should include the salient features of both history and examination: e.g. 74-year-old retired plumber with a 24 hour history of chest pain and breathlessness. On examination there were features of congestive cardiac failure which could be secondary to a myocardial infarction.

Provisional or differential diagnosis (or 'Problem list', see p. 63)

This should be written out in the true sequence of events, thus:

1. The aetiology
2. The pathological process
3. The structural lesion (if any)
4. Disorder of function (if any)

E.g. Chronic rheumatic carditis, mitral stenosis, atrial fibrillation, cardiac failure.

Special investigations

The results of special investigations should be included in the progress notes and, when any large series of investigations is made, e.g. serial blood counts, erythrocyte sedimentation rates or examination of the cerebrospinal fluid, the results should be expressed by a graph on squared paper or on a flow sheet.

You should write brief progress notes on your patients every day. Documentation that the condition has not changed may be just as important as recording changes in condition.

Operation notes (where indicated)

If you attended the operation make your own notes, but if not summarise the official operation notes.

Discharge note

A full statement of the patient's condition on discharge should be written and a note made of his/her destination (e.g. home, convalescent home, other hospital. Recommended after-care should be noted, and an estimate made of the prognosis. If the patient dies, you should attend the post-mortem and then complete his/her notes by a short account of the autopsy findings.

Final diagnosis (or 'Final problem list', see p. 70)

The final diagnosis reached at the time of discharge, or as confirmed by post-mortem, must be given in every case.

63

Problem orientated medical record (POMR)

Problem orientated medical records (POMR) differ little from conventional records apart from laying great emphasis on the construction of a complete list of the patient's problems. Their major attributes are that they ensure that problems and the follow-up of problems are not forgotten and that the information contained in them is more readily computerised. This account will simply outline the principles of constructing such records. (For full account see L.L. Weed (1968). Medical records that guide and teach. *New England Journal of Medicine*, *278*, 593 and 652.)
The record has four parts:

1. Data base
2. Problem list
3. Initial plans
4. Follow-up notes

1. Data base

This is the conventional record of the history and examination, plus any available investigations.

2. Problem list

This is a complete list of *all* the patient's problems (separated into active problems and inactive problems) derived from the history and examination and from the results of investigations. Each problem is given a number, its date of entry is recorded and the list is then placed at the front of the notes (see 'Case illustration', p. 65).

Problems may be:

Precise diagnoses

Pathophysiological states, such as cardiac or respiratory failure

Symptoms, abnormal physical signs, and abnormal investigation results which are not encompassed by a disease or syndrome already on the list

Psychiatric problems

Social problems

Risk factors

Past illnesses

64

They should be statements of fact, not hypotheses, or guesses, and should be stated at the highest level compatible with the facts and your understanding of them. If a patient has abdominal pain and you do not know the cause, then 'abdominal pain' is the title of the problem; if you have good evidence that the pain is due to duodenal ulcer then 'duodenal ulcer' is the title of the problem.

3. Initial plans

Having identified and recorded the problems the POMR system then considers *each active problem* separately under the following headings, and a statement about each is recorded where appropriate.

> **Goal** (e.g. level to which blood pressure is to be lowered)
> **Diagnostic information required** (i.e. list of diagnostic tests necessary)
> **Monitoring required** (i.e. the physical measurements or serial laboratory tests required)
> **Treatment** (this includes all forms of treatment, not just drug therapy)
> **Patient education** (this includes a statement about what the patient and/or a relative is told about his/her condition and instruction about practical procedures – for example, that a diabetic patient has been taught to draw up and inject insulin, to care for the syringe and to test the urine)

4. Follow-up notes

These are essentially the same as in the conventional system except that the POMR considers *each active problem* separately under the following headings:

> **Changes in symptoms**
> **Changes in physical signs or the results of investigations**
> **Re-assessment of the problem in the light of the above** (this may enable a vague problem title to be changed to a more precise title, e.g. 'abdominal pain' to 'duodenal ulcer'; and the problem list is amended accordingly)
> **Further plans** (which are treated in the same way as 'initial plans')

65

Case illustration

19.7.83
Mr R. Jones, 1 Florence Way, Cambridge. Age 56. A baker.
Admitted as an emergency at 4.00 p.m. on 19.7.83 under the care
of Dr Z.

     c/o 1. Chest pains for three weeks
         2. Shortness of breath for two days

History of the present complaint

Perfectly fit and well until *three weeks ago* when he began to feel
rather unwell and to suffer episodic retrosternal chest pains which
were dull in character and radiated into his throat. Never very
severe. Tended to come on after the evening meal and also when
he was travelling to work by bike. Each bout lasted 15–30
minutes. Had one severe bout *ten days ago* lasting all evening and
keeping him awake until the early morning. *Since then* has had
one further episode of pain. Possibly related to exertion but
unaffected by posture or breathing and unrelieved by milk or
Rennies. Not associated with breathlessness or sweating. *Two
days ago*, noticed that he could not climb the stairs without stop-
ping for breath. Breathlessness has increased since then and he
now feels breathless at rest. Slight ankle swelling in the *last few
days*. Mild non-productive cough for *one week*. No wheeze, no
palpitations.

Past medical history

    General health good
    1960 (aet 38) Duodenal ulcer confirmed by barium meal.
      Hospitalised
      Trouble for two years but then symptom-free until now
    No diabetes, rheumatic fever or tuberculosis
    No jaundice. No operations

No diabetes, heart disease or peptic ulceration

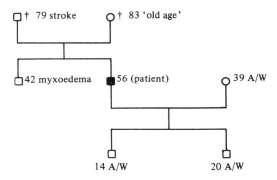

Social history

    Baker for 30 years – flour dust + +
    Smokes 25 cigarettes per day, alcohol socially only
    Lives with wife and two sons in their own home
    No social or financial problems

Drugs and allergy history

    Allergic to penicillin (came out in a rash when given
       penicillin for a sore throat)
    No other allergies
    No medication other than Rennies

Functional enquiry

    General health good. Sleeps well. No weight loss
CVS As above
RS As above
AS Appetite good
    No nausea or vomiting
    No abdominal pains
    No dysphagia. No acid regurgitation or heartburn
    Bowels open regularly × 1 daily. Normal faeces
GUS No dysuria, nocturia or frequency. Good stream
    No haematuria

67

CNS No headaches
No fits or faints
Vision normal. Hearing normal
No dizziness
No weaknesses or paraesthesiae
Right handed
Joints No back pains, joint or muscle pains

Physical examination

Gen: Looks unwell. Temperature 37.8 °C
Overweight
No pallor, cyanosis, jaundice or dehydration
No lymphadenopathy. No clubbing
Thyroid normal

CVS: Pulse 96 per minute, regular, normal character
JVP raised 8 cm. Ankle oedema to mid calf. No calf
    tenderness
No varicose veins
Blood pressure (right) lying 140/85
Apex beat – 6th intercostal space, 12 cm from midline,
    normal impulse
First and second HS normal. Third HS present. No
    murmurs
Peripheral pulses all present and equal

RS: Short of breath at rest, rate 26 per minute
Shape normal
Movements equal but poor expansion
Trachea central
Percussion note dull at both bases
Bilateral basal crackles (coarse)

AS: Mouth normal
Liver palpable 4 cm below costal margin:
    – smooth and tender
    – upper border of liver normal on percussion
Not distended, soft
No masses or tenderness
Spleen and kidneys not palpable
Hernial orifices intact
Genitalia normal
PR deferred

CNS: Alert and co-operative
Fundi normal
Rest of examination deferred until patient's condition
    improves

68

Subsequent analysis by POMR system

Problem list

(listed in the follow-up notes and also on a form ('final problem list') to be placed at the front of the notes)

Retrosternal chest pain – myocardial infarction
Shortness of breath
Ankle oedema
Cough
Basal crackles
Enlarged heart   Congestive cardiac failure
Raised JVP, 3rd HS
Enlarged liver
Obesity
Pyrexia
P.H. of duodenal ulcer
F.H. of stroke and hypertension
Allergy to penicillin
Smokes 25/day

Initial investigations

Haemoglobin (Hb) 15.2 g/dl. White blood cell count
  (WBC) 12.2×10^9/l
Urea and electrolytes normal
Chest X-ray (XR) – enlarged heart
  pulmonary oedema with small basal effusions
Electrocardiogram (ECG) – recent inferior myocardial
  infarction

Initial plans

1. *Myocardial infarction*
Diagnostic information – daily cardiac enzymes and ECG $\times$ 3

2. *Congestive cardiac failure*

Monitoring   – 4-hourly pulse and BP
                Examine daily for JVP, pulmonary oedema
                Fluid input/output chart
                Urea and electrolytes daily
                ECG monitor

Treatment	– Bed rest Diet – sodium restriction Frusemide 40 mg i.v. stat., thereafter Frusemide 40 mg and Triamterene 100 mg b.d. orally
Patient education	– Frightened by shortness of breath Told he has some fluid in his lungs because of heart attack and that this will respond to treatment

3. *Pyrexia*

Diagnostic
information
	– Probably secondary to the myocardial
	infarction but possible chest infection:
	   blood cultures × 3
	   sputum cultures × 3
	   CXR etc.
	?developing deep venous thrombosis (DVT)
	Check calves daily

4. *Obesity*

Goal	– Reach 68 kg within six months
Monitoring	– Weigh weekly in hospital
Treatment	– 1000 calorie diet – may need reducing diet later
Patient education	– Told of hazards of obesity, necessity of adher- ing to diet

FINAL PROBLEM LIST		Hospital No.	
		Surname	M / F
		First Names	M / S / W
		D. of B.	

PROBLEM NUMBER	I.C.D. No.	ACTIVE PROBLEMS Include Symptoms, Signs and Abnormal Investigations not Explained by Another Entry. Social and Psychiatric Problems Should Also Be Included.	DATE ENTERED	INACTIVE PROBLEMS Include Major Past Illness, Operations or Hypersensitivities. Do Not Include Problems for Which You Will Provide Active Care.
1		INFERIOR MYOCARDIAL INFARCT	19 : 7 : 83	
2		CONGESTIVE CARDIAC FAILURE (2° to (1)	19 : 7 : 83	
3		PYREXIA AND RAISED WBC	19 : 7 : 83	
4		OBESITY (weight 84 Kg)	19 : 7 : 83	
5		SMOKES 25 CIGS PER DAY	19 : 7 : 83	
6				DUODENAL ULCER (Age 40)
7				F.H. STROKE, HYPERTENSION
8				ALLERGY TO PENICILLIN
9				
10				
11				
12				
13				
14				
15				

71

Checklist for history and examination

History

c/o	(Complains of)
HPC	(History of the present complaint)
PMH	(Past medical history)
FH	(Family history)
PH and SH	(Personal and social history)
Drugs and allergy history	
FE	(Functional enquiry: minimal enquiry)

General
  Fatigue/malaise
  Sleep disturbance
  Weight loss or gain
  Skin rashes
CVS
  SOB
  Chest pain
  Palpitation
  Ankle swelling
RS
  SOB
  Chest pain
  Cough
  Wheezing
  Sputum
  Haemoptysis
AS
  Appetite/weight
  Bowels
  Nausea/vomiting
  Abdominal pain

GUS
  Micturition
  Prostatic symptoms
  Nocturia
  Haematuria
Menstruation
  Age at onset
  Menopause
  Length of period
  Periodicity
  Regularity
  Light or heavy
  Dysmenorrhoea
CNS
  Headache
  Fits/faints/dizziness
  Vision
  Hearing
  Weakness
  Numbness/paraesthesiae
  Anxiety/depression
Joints
  Pain, swelling, stiffness

72

Examination

Temp. Anaemia. Cyanosis. Jaundice. Clubbing
Lymphadenopathy. Breasts, Thyroid
CVS: Pulse. BP. JVP. Apex beat. Impulses. HS. Murmurs.
    Oedema
RS: Trachea. Shape. Movements. PN. TVF. BS. Added sounds
AS: Mouth. Abdominal tenderness.
    Liver/spleen/kidneys/masses. Hernial orifices. PR
CNS: Conscious level. Cranial nerves. Always specify fundi
    Limb tone/power/reflexes
Joints: If relevant